THE RISE AND FALL OF RHEUMATOID ARTHRITIS

THE RISE AND FALL OF RHEUMATOID ARTHRITIS

THE ROOT CAUSE OF RHEUMATOID ARTHRITIS IS...........

BY GEORGE "JACK" IRETON

Library of Congress Control Number:		2014904206
ISBN:	Hardcover	978-1-4931-8139-1
	Softcover	978-1-4931-8140-7
	eBook	978-1-4931-8138-4

In writing of this book, my thoughts and conclusions are my own and not of any physician, hospital or any other medical organization. All of the new ideas and any mistakes are mine. Hopefully, there will be a lot of the former and none of the latter.

This book was printed in the United States of America.

Rev. date: 03/03/2014

To order additional copies of this book, contact:
Xlibris LLC
1-888-795-4274
www.Xlibris.com
Orders@Xlibris.com
609409

CONTENTS

Dedication

This book is dedicated to my wife Doree, my sons and daughters and their families. You are my wealth and my inspiration in all that I do. Thank you for being you.

Also, this book is dedicated to my paternal grandmother, Florence Johnson Ireton, who I am sure, had R A and to about 2 Million people in the U.S. that fight the good fight against Rheumatoid Arthritis. The battle has been won.

ACKNOWLEDGEMENTS

A big thank you goes out to Bud Simpson, Author and Naturalist from Hocking County, Ohio for his tremendous guidance and editing help in putting this book together. I doubt that I would have completed it by myself. I was stuck in compound low gear and headed up a very steep hill.

FOREWORD

Vitamin deficiencies can be the cause of many health problems. I'm only a layman, but even I know that little fact. When I was a child, back in the late 1940's, I had severe nose bleeds for nearly all of one summer. Because of these nose bleeds, I spent more of that summer in the house than I did outside doing all the things a child should be able to do. In later years, a doctor told me that the nose bleeds were probably caused by a lack of Vitamin K.

In undeveloped countries, especially in Africa, blindness is a common, very dangerous, problem. It usually starts as night blindness but can escalate into total blindness and even eventual death. The cause in many cases? Vitamin A deficiency.

Until the 1980's, stomach ulcers were thought to be caused by stress, hot foods, fatty foods or acidic foods. Today, most stomach ulcers are generally thought to be caused by the bacterium; H. pylori. That's not a vitamin but I use it as an example to show that common thought may be wrong. Scientists can be wrong. Doctors can be wrong. Treatments for disease can be wrong.

I'm not endorsing the views of this book. All I'm saying is that the material contained herein deserves a good look. The author's theories about the root cause of Rheumatoid Arthritis, RA, deserve it.

Bud Simpson, Logan, Ohio

Bud Simpson is the author of two books—
"MANTAWASSUK: THE COVE" and his latest,
"THE MOVING FINGER WRITES".

THE PREFACE

Right at the beginning, I'd like you to know that I am not a Physician and have no medical agenda. I am not connected with any drug company. I am a retired Engineer after spending 40 years in the manufacturing industry. I am a first time author with no previous book publication experience. However, Engineers do have communications skills in a variety of technical areas. We will see if those skills carry over to being an author. You the reader will have to decide whether this is true or not.

In my life time, I have had several diseases that are now treated with childhood shots,—German measles, chicken pox, rubella, and whooping cough. I have been vaccinated for small pox several times. Also, thru the first 20+ years of my life, everyone was scared to death of Polio until that was overcome. Now that I have spent the last 26+ years with Rheumatoid Arthritis, I can say that I have successfully weathered that storm also.

In the early 1960's, President John Kennedy challenged NASA and the American people to "Put a man on the moon and return him safely to earth in this decade." That was done in 1969 to complete his vision. Here is my challenge to the Rheumatologists and Physicians in the United States. Control Rheumatoid Arthritis completely before the end of this decade. Before we hear a call go out to "lock up Grandpa before he falls into the deep end of the swimming pool", read on. You might be surprised at how easy it will be to do just that.

My qualification in writing about Rheumatoid Arthritis is that I have lived with it for over 26 years. Also, I have found the answer to this basic question, "What is the root cause of Rheumatoid Arthritis?" As I worked thru this scenario, I became my own test laboratory. My family was not too enthused about this approach as they were inclined to keep the status quo, which had been working, even though I was losing ground to RA.

There was no magic wand waving or new medical discovery because that's not my field. This book is an assembly of two facts, one was well known and the other was a little obscured and along with my experience. It is a quick read but as we would say about an offensive lineman in football, it's beefy. This book is meant to be a reference to a better life with RA under control.

I want to assure the current Rheumatoid Arthritis sufferers that a better way has been found to control this disease. It is based on attacking the cause and not the effect of Rheumatoid Arthritis which we have had to do for many generations. I have written this to relate my experiences that occurred over about 7 months in 2013 and will describe the events just as they unfolded.

After reading this book, you should consult your Physician about this approach and relate them to your own situation. I cannot be your doctor. I can only present to you what I have done and let you make your own healthcare determination. You are the only one that can do that. Cheer up. It will probably be the best decision of your adult life.

PROLOGUE

Rheumatoid Arthritis is a disease that inflames the joints of 1.5 to 2 million people in the U.S. alone. If the RA is not treated, it can become very painful and can debilitate the patient. Of the RA patients, 75 to 80 % are woman who have suffered a lot more than this male author did. It hits the ladies harder and more frequently. As we will learn later, this is may be do due to occupation and/ or exposure and obviously to gender. Also, as we age, our bodies do not process normal functions as well as we did when we were younger. This is apparent since both male and female develop RA more during their mid adult years. My RA was diagnosed when I turned 51.

As we will learn later, RA is treatable, reversible and should be preventable. Also, there are strong facts that certain chemicals we inhale on a day to day basis cause the condition that leads to RA. That is a lot of strong words from a non-medical person about such an important medical subject. So let us begin to sort this out.

CHAPTER 1

In the early 1980's, I received a preview of coming attractions with a round with "tennis shoulder" and other aches and pains associated with the beginning of Rheumatoid Arthritis. These were nagging type of pains that were treated with drugs that worked on the effect (after the fact) and only provided temporary relief. Finally, in 1987, I was diagnosed with RA. The next 18 months were pretty much miserable with the RA winning the battle.

One of the biggest challenges during this period was trying to get enough rest. My fatigue and loss of sleep were so bad that I went on sleep medication which I had not had to do before or since. If I could manage 5 hours of sleep, I considered that as having a good night.

In the fall of 1988, I was referred to the RA clinic at The Ohio State University. My Sedimentation Rate (commonly known as sed rate, a term which most RA patients are familiar with) in consecutive months was 129 and 145 mm/hr. where the normal limits for my age then were 0-20. Needless to say that I was having a hard time getting out of a chair but I continued with a full time job in an industrial plant.

CHAPTER 2

Methotrexate

In January 1989, my whole life changed with the introduction of Methotrexate, a chemotherapy drug that kills cancer cells. When used against RA, it suppresses the immune system to keep down the joint inflammation. A depressed immune system is not all that good a thing considering that any future infections that the patient would develop would be hard to fight with the immune system in a depressed state. That would put you between a rock and a hard place. The immune system needs to be strong to fight infection and, at the same time, needs to be suppressed to control RA.

The Physician at the clinic slowly worked my dosage up to 6 Methotrexate tablets @ 2.5 mg each weekly. When I reached this magic dosage, it was as if I had "fallen off of a table" because the change was so sudden. I had been given my life back. I could actually function almost normally. What a relief!

Over the next 24 + years, to keep the same quality of life, I had to slowly increase the dosage of Methotrexate to 9.5-2.5mg tablets per week. I averaged over 8 tablets per week for 24 years+ or over 10,000 Methotrexate tablets totally!

The disease was slowly winning because I was approaching the max allowable dosage of 10-2.5 mg or 25 mg of Methotrexate weekly just to stay even with the disease with no improvement. The history of RA has shown that at some point in time, the Methotrexate alone would not be effective or could not be tolerated and you must move on to other treatments or combinations of treatments and, definitely, to a lesser lifestyle.

I was reaching a point much like the story that Mark Twain wrote in the 1897 travel book "Following the Equator: A Journey Around the World". This story was about a woman whose health was failing. He wrote the following:

"She had run down and down and down, and had at last reached a point where medicines no longer had any helpful effect upon her. I said I knew I could put her upon her feet in a week. It brightened her up, it filled her with hope, and she said she would do everything I told her to do. So I said she must stop swearing and drinking, and smoking and eating for four days, and then she would be all right again.

"And it would have happened just so, I know it; but she said she could not stop swearing, and smoking and drinking, because she had never done those things. So there it was. She had neglected her habits, and hadn't any. Now that they would have come good, there were none in stock. She had nothing to fall back on. She was a sinking vessel, with no freight in her to throw overboard and lighten ship withal."

Every RA patient, sooner or later, comes to the same conclusion. What are we supposed to throw overboard to keep our ship from sinking? What we really need is to patch the hole so the ship won't sink. The Methotrexate plug that we stuck in that leaky ship 24 years ago was about as large now as we could make it, while the hole caused by RA was getting larger still. Our attempts to close the hole were not working and our ship was slowly sinking. Also, my Methotrexate dose was fast approaching toxic levels.

NSAID FELDENE

The first drug that I was started on in 1987 to combat the RA was the NSAID (non-steroidal, anti-inflammatory, drug) Feldene. It alone did not contain the RA but it battled alone until the right medication was found.

By late in 2012, I had consumed over 9300-20 mg tablets or 186,000 mg of generic Feldene to go with all of the Methotrexate. In 2012, my Physician had been encouraging me to quit using NSAIDs because of their potential bad reaction in the digestive system. It was time to get off this medication. So, at the end of 2012 and the first 3 months of 2013, I managed to partially get off of the use of NSAIDs. I say partially because I was still having to "fall off the wagon" every week to ten days. I could not entirely shake the need because the Methotrexate alone was not doing the job of containing and reducing the joint inflammation and back pain.

CHAPTER THREE

Dawn Of A New RA Era

VITAMIN D

During my semiannual visit with my Physician on March 10, 2013, we discussed my lack of energy. He proposed that as a part of my blood work, the lab would run a test on level of Vitamin D. As I learned later, Vitamin D is responsible for several critical operations in body. It is the one and only guardian of the joints against inflammation. A low Vitamin D level leads to joint inflammation.

In the meantime, while I waited on the lab results, I started to take an additional 1000 IU of Vitamin D3 along with the 600 IU from the multivitamin I had been taking for some time. That made a total of 1600 IU of Vitamin D3 I consumed daily.

My physician told me "not to feel like the Lone Ranger. Lots and lots of RA patients have taken Vitamin D. Don't think that you are breaking new ground". Even with that pronouncement, I had to pursue Vitamin D full steam ahead. There was no other answer.

As it turned out, of all my blood work, the Vitamin D level was the only criteria out of its acceptable specification range. Vitamin D 25-Hydroxy, which is the fancy name for the test, was 35.5 ng/ml. A normal range would be considered 30-100 and a medium or good range of 50-60. When the results came back, the Doctor raised my Vitamin D3 level by 1000 IU to 2600 IU per day.

The immediate result was spectacular in that I no longer felt the need for the weekly NSAID to combat joint inflammation. Wow! Want to run that by me again? I no longer felt the need for the occasional NSAID to combat joint inflammation. Would the Vitamin D deficiency be the root cause of RA? The NSAID was definitively working on the effect. Both the NSAID and the Methotrexate act after the fact on RA. Would the Methotrexate, which also works on the effect of RA, be necessary if the right dosage of Vitamin D, which appeared to work on the cause, was obtained? If that is true, then RA could be a reversible disease. And, if it's reversible, why would it not be preventable? Over the next 10 weeks, I set out to investigate all of the above. That might be the news that I had been waiting on for 26 years!

So if I can't be that other guy, the Lone Ranger, then, "Ernie the RA Engineer" would have to ride out and find out all about this Vitamin D dude and put a rope on him and any faithful companion.

The only way to prove the case for not needing Methotrexate to control RA would be to slowly and carefully back off the dosage of 9.5-2.5 mg tablets while slowly raising the Vitamin D3.

So on to the one and only Case Study associated with this investigation.

CHAPTER 4

Case study on the effect of Vitamin D3 on Rheumatoid Arthritis

Objective: To determine if there was a level of Vitamin D3 intake that would allow the total withdrawal of Methotrexate.

Sample size	1
Patients name	George Ireton.*
Study conducted by	George Ireton
Patients age at the diagnosis of RA	51
Number of years on Feldene, (NSAID)	26 (1987 till March 2013)
Number of years on Methotrexate	24 (Jan. 1989 till?)
Drug used in study	Vitamin D3 gels (O.T.C.)
Start date	March 2013.

Dosage of Vitamin D3

2600 UI per day at meals (Mar-Apr. 2013)

3600 UI per day, divided among 3 meals (May 1, 2013)

4600 UI per day, divided among 3 meals and snack. (May 15, 2013)

5600 UI per day, divided among 3 meals and snack. (May 22, 2013)

6600 UI per day, divided among 3 meals. (May 27, 2013)

8600 UI per day, divided among 3 meals + snack.
(June 19, 2013)

Medical history

Patient was diagnosed with Type II Diabetes in 2003. Patient controlled the Diabetes by losing weight and by diet.

Cholesterol has never been a problem.

Allergies (pine needles), colds other respiratory illnesses have been controlled very effectively with a large daily dose of Vitamin C— (1500 mg).

* Patients name and medical data used with permission of Patient.

Procedure: Slowly decrease the weekly dosage of Methotrexate. Evaluate each step week by week. When discomfort level increases, the dosage of Vitamin D3 would be increased to a higher level. Having to back track to higher level of Methotrexate would be to abort the test.

The following is the weekly tracking of the decrease in Methotrexate dosage:

Week 1 March 24, 2013	Decrease the dosage to 9.0 tablets
Week 2 March 31, 2013	Dosage remained at 9.0 tablets.
Week 3 April 7, 2013	Decrease the dosage to 8.5 tablets
Week 4 April 14, 2013	Dosage remained at 8.5 tablets
Week 5 April 21, 2013	Decrease the dosage to 8.0 tablets

Week 6 April 28, 2013	Decrease the dosage to 7.5 tablets
Week 7 May 5, 2013	Decrease the dosage to 6.5 tablets
Week 8 May 12, 2013	Decrease the dosage to 5.5 tablets
Week 9 May 19, 2013	Decrease the dosage to 0. *

*The initial level of relief in 1989 when I first started Methotrexate treatment was 6 tablets of 2.5 mg each weekly. Once I reached the level of 5.5 tablets and remained there for a week, which was 42% below the initial starting point, it would be apparent at that point in time that the Methotrexate was no longer necessary and I could safely take the final step of going to the 0 dosage level at the start of week 9.

Results:

First weeks: Caution! Proceed very slowly.

Middle weeks: Proceed more aggressively by decreasing a pill a week. Increase the Vitamin D3 dosage to compensate for the loss of Methotrexate.

End: 6.5 to 5.5 pills a week was a big move since that dropped me below the initial level that gave me relief in 1989.

The grand end: The next week, I stopped taking any Methotrexate! Imagine the excitement and relief. I could go ahead with the knowledge that I was not dependent on the high potency drug Methotrexate to work on the effect of Rheumatoid Arthritis rather than the root cause of Rheumatoid Arthritis which is Vitamin D deficiency. Let us repeat that again.

The root cause of Rheumatoid Arthritis is Vitamin D deficiency.

Even after this discovery, there was something missing. Something was not quite right. I was experiencing muscle cramps and not doing the stairs well. So it was back to the Search Engine, since there are not a lot of drawing boards that I can go back to now as the old saying goes.

CHAPTER 5

Companion Mineral

During one of my sessions in my favorite text book, the internet, I found a reference to link Vitamin D and the mineral Magnesium. In an article on the Livestrong.com on Aug. 18, 2011, Owen Bond, nutritionist, stated the following:

"IT (Magnesium) is also required by all the enzymes that metabolize vitamin D. Initial symptoms of magnesium deficiency include muscle cramps, which are often exacerbated by sunbathing because large amounts of vitamin D are produced within the skin in response to sunlight and deplete magnesium levels even further. Supplementing with vitamin D can also exacerbate an underlying magnesium deficiency.

From this, we can conclude that Vitamin D blood levels will fail to rise in those who are already Magnesium deficient, irrespective of their vitamin D consumption. **Let us hit this again**. So, taking large dosages of Vitamin D alone, which is the current medical practice, is counterproductive if the patient is deficient in Magnesium or if you're not adding sufficient Magnesium to balance the increase in Vitamin D. This is the reason that I struggled for the first 10 weeks of taking Vitamin D alone without adding Magnesium. And what are the chances that a large number of RA patients are deficient in Magnesium? The probability is very high, possibly 90% or greater.

Also, according to the article, Magnesium relieves muscle cramps, along with several other things. When cramping occurs, it is generally attributed, incorrectly, to an overdose of Vitamin D, like you feel after a long day at the beach, instead of the real reason which is Magnesium deficiency.

Well, now Dude, we are talking about real facts that we can throw a rope around. The down side of Magnesium is that it is contained in nuts and leafy greens. How big a pile of leafy greens would this meat and potatoes guy have to eat that would be needed to balance a daily intake of 8600 IU of Vitamin D? Could I actually see over such a pile? It might be as tall as our 16 year old grandson. That thought was terrifying to contemplate. I immediately headed for my friendly grocery pharmacy to see what Magnesium was available OTC (over the counter).

The Magnesium, in the form of Magnesium Oxide, was listed on the bottle as a dietary supplement. The recommended dosage was 3 large "horse pills" a day with meals for a total of 400 mg of Magnesium, per day. Good place to start. After a day or two at that dosage, with not much improvement, I doubled the dosage to 6 pills which is 800 mg per day. One week later, I adjusted it to 1200 mg per day and in June to 1600 mg per day. Later on in 2013, I scaled back to 1067 mg per day to a balance of 1000IU of

Vitamin D3 for every 133 mg of Magnesium. This is self-regulating since taking too much Magnesium acts as a laxative. Remember the product called Milk of Magnesia? The Magnesium tablets are large but tasteless.

BINGO! Does that feel good or what! I have been transported back 30 years to "Before RA ". As the color analyst for Monday night Football sang when the game became out of reach, "Turn out the lights. The party's over". And the party is really over for RA because now *__The root cause of Rheumatoid Arthritis is a deficiency in Vitamin D AND a deficiency in Magnesium__*. You can't have one without the other. "The root cause of Rheumatoid Arthritis is a deficiency in Vitamin D AND a deficiency Magnesium". It sounds like we have a winner.

The human body has a ph. range of 7.35-7.45, which is slightly basic. Soft drinks with a ph. in the low 6's, is acidic. Magnesium with a ph. of 10.3 is more than slightly basic. If you drink a soft drink while you eat lunch, and you intend to take Magnesium with Vitamin D, the soft drink may react with the Magnesium causing it to be less effective with the Vitamin D. Isn't that a bummer! There goes my diet cola at meal time. In fact, now I wait a while after meals before starting the next cola.

I know that someone will question whether I still have RA. I have no muscle cramping which is a biggie. I am still able to go up and down the three sets of stairs in our house as I did 40 years ago. That was beginning to be a problem with Vitamin D alone. My RA is now totally controlled. And everyone else who has RA can do the same thing because we are now treating the cause not the effect of RA. All of the former treatments for the effects of RA, which include Methotrexate, have been eliminated.

Plus and Minuses

Large pluses: The elimination of Methotrexate and all of the bad baggage that comes with that chemotherapy drug. That would include possible liver damage, skin cancer and the beat down feeling that comes once a week when your blood cells are attacked.

The other real "biggie" is reversal of hair loss. I have managed to regrow a decent amount of hair on several square inches of my scalp. Although the gain is small, it is in the right direction. Chemo drugs do a number on hair.

Small pluses include better looking and feeling finger and toe nails. It was very evident as I watched the toe nails grow out over a 6 month period and completely change in color and texture. Second, this winter, I did not experience dry cracked hands as I have for as long as I can remember. It may be happenstance and may take several winters to prove out that theory.

Minuses: There are none. Some people might consider the large size and quantity of the Magnesium pills to be a challenge. That is a minor inconvenience considering the gain. If the pills are giving you a problem in swallowing, break them in half. One way or the other, the Magnesium is needed to metabolize the Vitamin D.

CHAPTER 6

The Probable Cause of the Root Cause of Rheumatoid Arthritis is . . . . the Inhalation of Volatile Organic Compounds, commonly shortened to V.O.C. These chemicals deplete the Vitamin D in the blood stream in the lungs.

The EPA definition of a Volatile Organic Compound is a "chemical that is photo chemically reactive" which means that the chemical reacts with sunlight to form smog. RA patients are only concerned with the effect that these compounds have when we breathe them and have to deal with the effects on our lungs.

Here are at least four causes of the root cause of Rheumatoid Arthritis:

1. Paint solvents
2. Ammonia from pet urine, baby's diapers, and litter boxes
3. Gasoline vapors
4. Chlorine bleach and swimming pool chlorine

PAINT SOLVENTS

My contention has been from day 1 in 1987 that my exposure to paint solvents both at work and at home was the basic cause for my RA. At home, we have been working on our old white farm house for 40 years. In the past, I have joked that the first 100 gallon of paint and varnish that we applied were the hardest. I am sure that we have long since passed the 100 gallon mark. Couple that with my in-door job where I did not get a lot of sunshine and my contact with industrial painting processes, led to the high probability that inhalation of paint solvents caused RA.

Until the discovery of the tie in between Vitamin D and Magnesium, it did not become apparent that the decrease in Vitamin D in my blood stream came thru the lungs. For 26 years, paint solvents would set off a RA episode which means that I would develop extreme joint inflammation in 24 to 36 hours after inhalation exposure. Vitamin D is the necessary and is the lone inflammation fighter in the cells of the joints. If the Vitamin D is low, the inflammation goes up and thus an RA is created.

AMMONIA

Ammonia made the list when we happened to meet a lady that ran a kennel where we picked up a new pup. The woman had a very severe case of RA. She was constantly exposed to dog urine in her kennel area which contained a very high concentration of Ammonia. Afterward, I received an RA episode in the usual 24 to 36 hours. The woman was constantly being bombarded by the ammonia fumes that attacked the Vitamin D in her blood stream via the lungs. It would be hard to estimate how much Vitamin D and Magnesium that she would have to take to overcome that constant ammonia attack. She might have to walk away from the business to back track and cure her RA.

Other areas where ammonia comes into play are baby's diapers, cat litter boxes and probably at Veterinary Clinics which could contribute to the same problem as the kennel owner. Also, anyone with a long term exposure to ammonia as a cleaning solvent is apt to be a candidate for RA. However, this application of ammonia is not as common as it was previously.

GASOLINE

Gasoline makes the top 4 list due a couple of encounters that I had with it before Magnesium. These incidences were similar to the episode described in the ammonia section previously. In 24 to 36 hours after exposure, the RA hits hard for 24 hrs. +. In these 2 cases, the exposure came from changing the fuel filter on a gasoline engine. Without protection of adequate Vitamin D in my blood to fight the gasoline vapors attack, I suffered a RA episode that lasted at least 24 hours. Now, with the Vitamin D level in my blood at 60, I should not experience the same result.

CHLORINE

Chlorine made the list because of the wide usage as laundry bleach and as the primary pool water sanitizer. In both cases, care has to be exercised when handling them because each give off chlorine vapors, whether the Chlorine is in solid or liquid form. As my high school chemistry teacher said about Nitric Acid, which could include Chlorine: 1. Chlorine eats organic material. 2. You are organic material.

Chlorine is very aggressive against organic material. In its dilute form, Chlorine sanitizes our drinking water and our swimming pool water and it bleaches our laundry.

The inhalation of Chlorine has been considered very bad for a really long time. Chlorine gas was used as a weapon of war during WW I, with devastating effects due to the unpredictability of wind currents. The person using the weapon might incur as many casualties as the enemy!

CHAPTER 7

Muscle Cramps

I have been reminded on two occasions when I was using Vitamin D alone that vibration can bring on swollen joints and muscle cramps in hours. Those two occasions involve saws, an electric rotary saw and hand saw, both of which took about 24 hours in recovery time. The other saw action which has been a disaster for me to operate is a chain saw. These examples are mainly "guy things" but illustrate that vibration was not friendly to healthy joints.

Since I have been writing this from day one of the Vitamin D investigation, it reads partly as a journal. Let me update the part that magnesium plays in this interaction. Magnesium decreases muscle cramps especially when high dosages of Vitamin D are taken either through sunlight or supplement form. It was important to remember that I went 10 weeks before I discovered the need for increased magnesium in my diet. The muscle cramps that I receive from vibration are from Magnesium deficiency and not the vibration or high dosage of Vitamin D. I was able to test that theory soon after I established a program of Magnesium with Vitamin D. Muscle cramps are a thing of the past for me.

Let us expand this theory on muscle cramps to see how it applies to your favorite football team. It is an early September Saturday afternoon in the stadium. The weather forecast is for clear skies with temperatures in the high 80's. This kind of weather tests the staff and players to keep well hydrated in order to avoid muscle cramps.

That leads to the question of why do some players on teams or whole teams get muscle cramps and some not. During the game a player can take in as much as 150,000+ IU (International Units) of Vitamin D from the sun.

One theory that comes to mind is that football teams in the grind of September sun have a very important issue to deal with along with the basic dehydration. That issue is whether the players have enough Magnesium in their systems to keep a balance with the high intake of Vitamin D from sun. If not, this could explain why individual players on the same team and from one team to another are more prone to cramping. I can picture down the road when this link between muscle cramps and Magnesium is recognized, a football team's diet will include foods high in Magnesium and/or provide a Magnesium supplement. That would certainly help in the fight against muscle cramps.

CHAPTER 8

Vitamin Storage

I'd like to relate the Vitamin D storage to the storage of chlorine in a swimming pool. When the thousands of pool owners (By the way we have 10 million swimming pools in the US!) ready their pools for use in the spring, the main parameter they are looking for is to obtain and maintain is a "free chlorine" level in the pool water.

After adjusting the ph. to 7.2-7.6, it is time to add enough chlorine and algaecide to kill the organics in the water and to clear up any cloudiness that occurred over the winter. When a "free" Chlorine level is reached, the chlorine and algaecide have done their initial job. At this point, there remains an amount of free stabilized chlorine of 1-4 ppm in the water to take care of the organics that the swimmers contribute to the pool. To maintain the free chlorine level, the chlorine that is added from this time on along with a weekly dosage of algaecide needs to balance and stay ahead of the pool load. Maintaining the free chlorine level will keep the pool clear and safe to swim in.

Now let us relate this to Vitamin D control in the blood "pool" in the body. There are certain needs to be met by the Vitamin D before we can talk about storage. Those needs include bone maintenance and the whopping biggie of supplying the joint cells with enough Vitamin D to fight inflammation.

In order to fill up my blood pool with enough Vitamin D and Magnesium to bring both up to good levels, I had to consume over one Million IU (International Units) of Vitamin D3 and over 133,000 mgs of Magnesium. It took over 4 months to bring the Vitamin D level in my blood up to 60!! How many Units of Vitamin D went to "storage" in fat Tissue? (For clarification, Vitamin D is fat soluble while Vitamin C is water soluble. For this reason, Vitamin D3 should always be taken with meals.) Probably not many I'd guess. The average RA patient has a very deep depleted pool of Vitamin D and Magnesium. If you start into this program, don't expect it to be a quick fix because it takes time to "fill your pool". Now, that time could be shortened because originally I proceeded slowly in coming down with the Methotrexate dosage and adding the Magnesium. If you take 10,000 IU of D3 daily, it would take 100 days to reach 1,000,000 IU.

And what about a possible over dose of Vitamin D? At this point in time, which is 10 months after starting the D3 program, I have consumed about 2 million IU of Vitamin D3 and 267,000 mg of Magnesium. There are no signs of overdose. I now have total control over RA with natural ingredients acting on its root cause.

Since the need for Vitamin D is constant, it is hard to use the word "elimination" to describe the end result of taking Vitamin D for Rheumatoid Arthritis. A better term would be "controlled" like diabetes. This would appear to be a life time of monitoring and taking Vitamin D3, and Magnesium especially for persons living in regions where they receive little benefit from the Vitamin D supplied by the sun and/or people employed in certain occupations.

It is also very important to remember that when you run into "hiccups" in your evaluation of how much Vitamin D to take, you do not want to say "I need to go back on Methotrexate" or other treatments. Those drugs treat the effect of RA and only Vitamin D treats the cause of RA and controls it for a way better life style.

CHAPTER 9

Fingers

Let us dwell a minute on the fingers and why they are so susceptible to RA. The blood vessels leaving the heart are large and have high carrying capacity. As they progress further and further from the heart, they become smaller, with some of the smallest being found in the fingers. With a high surface area to mass ratio and small blood vessels, the fingers get cold rapidly in cold weather and require close fitting gloves to keep them warm.

Well duh, tell us something we don't already know! Ok, the only way that the Vitamin D gets transferred to the joints in the fingers is through the very small blood vessels in the hand. Consequently there is poor Vitamin D servicing of the hand, causing the joints to swell up sooner and more than any of the other joints. For that reason, finger joints are stiffest in the AM after a night's sleep because the fingers have not been exercised, which stimulates blood flow.

Also, your blood pressure is the highest when you wake up because the blood vessels are constricted during sleep which in turn causes poor circulation to the fingers and other joints. That is why it is extremely important to start exercising in the AM. A hot shower dilates the blood vessels and decreases blood pressure.

In Sept. 2013, over 4 months after getting off Methotrexate, my left hand started to give me a problem first with my ring finger swelling up. At the same time, that same wrist that held my watch band for 50 +years was tightening up. This was the beginning of classic Carpal Tunnel with the tingling in the three and a half fingers, especially the thumb.

Although my surgeon that operated on my Carpal Tunnel stated that there is no connection between my Carpal Tunnel and the circulation to my fingers, my hands feel better in the morning when I control the CT and the circulation with wrist braces at night.

CHAPTER 10

Prevention

We have seen that RA is treatable and reversible, let us now consider whether is preventable. The same reasoning that led us to the cause of RA is the same argument that I would use to say very definitely that RA is preventable. If we would start at about the age of 30 to 35 to monitor blood levels of Vitamin D and Magnesium, we should be able to prevent RA.

This is especially important for the ladies approaching menopause. If menopause creates a more aggressive action against the Vitamin D in the blood, that would explain why a lot more women than men have RA. That type of monitoring would take a large amount of effort but would be well worth it.

Let us visit the need for better, faster and cheaper Vitamin D blood monitoring system. The RA patient needs a better, quicker, inexpensive feedback on their Vitamin D levels. What we need is a finger stick from a drop of blood, much like diabetes, that would give us our Vitamin D reading. From now on, RA patients will only be concerned with "What is my Vitamin D level and is it high enough to keep my joints free of inflammation and pain"? That feedback needs to come as quickly and as often as diabetes, not a week from now and at a great expense. Most insurance Companies will pay for a test for Vitamin D only every 2-3 months. The RA Patient needs to have that test "on demand" and in a very economical form.

The Rheumatologists, who are now against a wall trying to treat the effects of RA, then, would have the tools to treat patients for the cause of RA with meaningful treatment and prevention in the case of non-RA patients.

How neat a thing would that be for the next generation to be able to completely eliminate Rheumatoid Arthritis? That should be our goal. Treat and reverse the existing patients and prevent the next generations from catching the disease. That would be a truly outstanding achievement.

CHAPTER 11

Summary

Fact number 1: The joints in the arms and legs depend on Vitamin D exclusively to fight joint inflammation.

Fact number 2: Vitamin D depends on Magnesium in a precise ratio to metabolize the Vitamin D so that it can be used in multiple ways in the body. My ratio is 133 mgs of Magnesium (in the form of one Magnesium oxide tablet) for each 1000 IU of Vitamin D3. In the 2 articles that I read on this ratio, both said the ratio existed but didn't detail it. If any reader knows what this precise ratio is, please e-mail it to me. It is one of the missing details in this analysis.

This ratio was strengthened when my Vitamin D blood report for the 3 months sampled on June 12, 2013 came back as 50.8 while taking 6000 IU of D3. My Magnesium was in the upper good mid-range. If we consider the beginning D blood reading on March 10, 2013 of 35.5 on 0 Vitamin D (Disregard the 600 IU in the multivitamin) and compare it with the June 12 reading of 50.8, the difference shows a change of approximately 15 points with the use of 6000 IU of Vitamin D. That calculates to a 2.5 point raise in the D blood level for every 1000 IU of D. If we extrapolate this to the present dosage of 8000 IU of D, that would give a reading of 55 which is dead center of the preferred range of 50-60.

Later when I had been taking 8000 IU per day of Vitamin D, my blood work of September 2013 showed a Vitamin D level of 62 which is outstanding. When my next blood level comes back in March 2014, I may be able to cut back on the amount of D3 and Magnesium in order to keep the D level between 55 and 60. I feel that at this level I can survive an exposure to any of 4 VOC's (paint solvents, ammonia, chlorine and gasoline) without creating a RA episode.

When discussing the right level of Vitamin D and Magnesium, consider the fact that it could take less of a quantity to stay at a Vitamin D blood level of 55-60 than was required to get there. It should follow Newton's law of motion that states that a body in motion tends to stay in motion. A body at rest tends to stay at rest. The energy that it takes to accelerate your car to 60 mph far exceeds the energy to keep it there. I should be able to cut back to 6000 or 7000 IU of Vitamin D per day and hold a blood level of 55-60.

Fact number 3: In evaluating the treatment of RA, we have to ensure that we don't try to apply the Vitamin D and Magnesium treatment to areas that are giving pain that are not related to RA. That would include the back and neck, nerve pain from Carpal Tunnel, ligament damage, osteoarthritis and sore muscles and anything else not associated with the arm and leg joints. It is too easy to lump all of your aches and pains in one category and blame the RA medications for not curing all your pains.

The other areas that may benefit from better servicing with Vitamin D are bones. However, Vitamin D cannot compensate for physical damage. Also you need to know what your Vitamin D and Magnesium levels are before you start your program so you have a base line.

CHAPTER 12

Epilogue

What is it like to be on Vitamin D and Magnesium instead of Methotrexate? During the day, the difference is very noticeable. My back has improved. The spinal column is technically not eligible to have RA but I am sure, can benefit from "bone repair" with higher concentrations of Vitamin D. That seems to be the case with me.

The bad side is there is still some stiffness in the morning. This is probably due to poor night time circulation and not constantly moving new Vitamin D to the Joints, especially the fingers. However, within 1 to 1 ½ hours of your first morning dose, with a hot shower and exercise, the night's stiffness is mostly gone.

Let us talk a little bit about Vitamin D2 vs. D3. D2 is the version prescribed by your physician in units of 10,000 per pill. It is given once per day or per week and is known to be less effective than D3. Its claim to fame is that is a purer form of D than D3. Since it is on prescription, there is co-pay involved. The D3 is OTC and is available in 1000, 2000 and 5000 IU. If I had to depend on D2 from my physician, this study could not have been completed because I would not have had the flexibility to pick and choose the right combination of Vitamin D and Magnesium.

And if you consider the risk of OTC Vitamin D and Magnesium, there is none. Both D3 and Magnesium are required by the body and in the case of middle aged adults and RA patients, in very large quantities. It is a win-win situation in that we can now replace the drugs that work on the effect of RA and are patient unfriendly with drugs that are friendly and natural and work on the cause. It doesn't get any better than that.

MEDICATIONS

What will happen to the injectable treatments for RA? There is no issue of whether to keep these drugs or not. They treat only the effect of RA not the cause of this terrible disease. Society is full of examples of items that come into being, have a life span and are gone.

The most recent example I can site involves the exhaust system on my car. In the last fifteen years, the exhaust systems on all vehicles have been converted from carbon steel that rusts out and has to be replaced every 2 1/2 to 3 years to stainless steel that does not need replacing for the life of the car. My car has a stainless exhaust system held in place by carbon steel clamps that rusted out. How dumb is that? That is like going to the dentist and having him tell you that the teeth are all good but the gums have to be replaced.

During the clamp replacement, I talked to owner of the exhaust repair shop about the fact that the clamps were made carbon steel and the exhaust system was made of stainless. He remarked that he was against the stainless steel systems because it was putting him out of the exhaust repair business. He had to convert to other auto repair operations to sustain his business. The exhaust repair business is an example of the evolution from one of poor product satisfaction to one of excellent satisfaction for the consumer. We don't have to be bothered with exhaust systems every 3 years or less. We don't have to think about it and we take it for granted.

Just like the carbon steel exhaust systems, the present RA drugs will stop being used. This will happen quickly because the RA patients will demand it.

SUPPLY

When the big push comes for Vitamin D and Magnesium, the drug companies will have to scramble to keep up with the demand for these products. Let us take my dosage for example and project it for 1,000,000 RA patients. For my daily dosage of 8600 IU of Vitamin D, I would require 8600IU per day x 365 days per year which equals 3.1 million units for one person. If that total is projected over 1,000,000 patients, the number goes to 3.1 trillion units or 3.1 billion 1000 IU pills! And this is on the low side considering the average Patient may require more than 8600 IU per day, at least initially, and the patient load could be considerably higher than 1,000,000. Likewise, for Magnesium, because of the extremely large pill size, the volume will be huge. All in all, I doubt that the drug companies are ready for that type of demand.

So, it appears that I had better lay in a one year supply of both before the rush begins. It will take that long for drug companies to catch up. Luckily, Vitamin D and Magnesium both have a shelf life between a 2 and 2.5 years.

WHAT IF

I have never been much of a person to look back on the past and do any amount of wishful thinking. However, in this case, I will allow this one transgression. If I had known 30 years what I know now about RA, I firmly believe that my quality of life would have been quite a bit higher. Neither the 10,000 Methotrexate nor the 9300 Feldene would have been consumed. I am truly fortunate that my liver has lasted this long to handle that load. My consolation is that neither my kids nor grandkids need suffer with RA.

CHAPTER 13

Stairs

Stairs have been an important part of our lives because our 100+ year old farm house has 3 flights. The 2 flights, from the basement to the first floor and from the second floor to the attic, have 10 steps each. From the first floor to the second are 14 steps. That makes the ceiling height on the first floor about 8'-6" and the ceiling height on the second floor about 7'-2".

You might ask why the big difference? Since the age of the house precludes me from talking to the builder, here is my speculation on what his thoughts might have been 100 years ago. If the builder had made the first floor to the ceiling 8'-0" and keeping the stair rise per step reasonable, he would have to make the number of steps to the second floor the unlucky 13. Bummer! He is not going to build a house with that stigma attached to it from the get go. That is the reason that this explanation ended up in unlucky Chapter 13.

Since I am a "numbers guy" instead of a "letters person" like my wife, I thought it would be fun to calculate how many steps, up and down stairs, I have taken in our 40 years of living here. If we take the average number of steps per flight as being 12, the average number of flights of stairs per day as 6, which is probably low, then I have taken 6 x 12 x 365 = 26,280 steps per year and 1,051,200 steps minimum in 40 years. That is really an over whelming number to comprehend.

And next you will ask why would you want to continue to go up and down so many stairs? As my physician stated, "stairs are good". I keep doing stairs so I can keep doing stairs and that will allow me to keep doing stairs. I had to find a way of curing RA so I could keep doing stairs. Maybe another ¼ million or so would be about right.

CHAPTER 14

Outside The Box Thoughts

IMMUNE DISEASES

Rheumatoid Arthritis has been considered an immune disease because the only way to treat it was to suppress the immune system. An over active immune system must have caused the RA and the only way to control it was to suppress it.

Let us look at this theory thru a different set of glasses. If we go back to the two examples in Bud Simpson's Foreword, both his childhood nose bleeds and the blindness in Africans were conditions, not diseases. There are no immunizations available to treat either other of these conditions like all of the other child hood diseases. Neither would be considered immune system diseases.

In this book, we have worked thru enough data to prove that RA follows a set of chemical laws in the body that dictate whether the joints are inflamed or not. It is not an immune disease just because the only way to treat RA was to suppress the immune system. RA was probably so named back in the time when everyone was totally at a loss as to what caused RA. Treating the effect and saying it relates to the cause is faulty reasoning. When the cause is treated, it is obvious that Rheumatoid Arthritis is a condition and not an immune disease.

I can't picture a "runaway" immune system indiscriminately causing RA. The body has to follow certain chemical laws. When the body is denied enough Vitamin D thru not enough sunshine or it is depleted in the lungs by common chemicals that we breathe, and/or we have insufficient intake of Magnesium, then joint inflammation develops. That is simple chemistry.

If this continues over time and the depletion of Vitamin D and Magnesium gets worse, the condition known as RA develops. Since this condition can be reversed by using Vitamins and minerals which are vital body components, how can this be an immune disease? Rheumatoid Arthritis is not an immune disease. It is a condition.

In the future, I wonder how many other immune diseases will be recognized as conditions and will be controlled like RA. Maybe RA's first cousin Lupus will be included, since it involves joint inflammation? I will leave that discussion for others as it is waaay above my pay grade.

CHAPTER 15

The Back Of The Book

This part involves one of my real big pet peeves. What time is it when someone prints or says 12 A.M.? Let's look at the definition of straight up 12 o'clock on standard time. When the clock reaches 12 o'clock straight up noon, the sun is at its highest point or zenith and is, theoretically, directly overhead, casting no shadows east and west. This is the definition of the Meridian. A.M. is an abbreviation for Anti-Meridian which comes from Latin word anti which means before and PM is the abbreviation for Post-Meridian where post is the Latin word for after. Since, by definition, 12 o'clock is the meridian, it is neither A.M. nor P.M. 12 o'clock is undefined as to AM and PM and it is undefined at midnight as to even what day it is.

On New Year's Eve, we celebrate the New Year at 12:00:00. But at this point, for one second, the month, day and year are all undefined. This can be extended to decades, centuries and millenniums also. On New Year's Eve 2000, which by definition, is the last year of the 1990s, the 20th century and the second millennium, (not 1999), for one second, time was undefined as to the month, day, year, decade, century and millennium! How neat is that! (A clarification is in order. Since a monk, way back in time, decided to start numbering our calendar with year 1 instead of year 0, all decades, centuries and millenniums must end with a 0 and not a 9.)

So if you write "12 AM", you are saying "Meridian before Meridian". Come again. Does this make any sense at all?

The military, long ago, solved this problem by using the 24 hour clock. If the time is written as 1200 hours, it is for certain that the reference is for the noon Meridian and not midnight. And conversely, if the time is stated as 2400 hours, it is read as midnight and not noon.

So the term 12 A.M. must go away because it is undefined and doesn't exist and has been long ago been replaced with military time or noon and midnight. Aren't you glad you read this far? I certainly feel better. "I took my Vitamin D and Magnesium at noon or 1200 hours" which indicates that you took your RA pills with your lunch at the Meridian. Congratulations! You're on your way to controlling your RA. Keep up the good work. You can do it!

And in parting, **GO BUCKS!**

George "Jack" Ireton 2014

Author can be contacted by E-mail.
Address: griley3@frontier.com